Land of Ice

I0223646

A. Sole

chipmunkapublishing
the mental health publisher

A. Sole

Published by
Chipmunkapublishing
PO Box 6872
Brentwood
Essex CM13 1ZT
United Kingdom

http://www.chipmunkapublishing.com

Chipmunkapublishing gratefully acknowledge the support of Arts Council England.

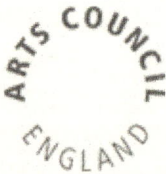

Author Biography

My name is A.Sole, I was born in Berlin on January seventh 1978. I have moved around constantly my whole life and have lived in as many as twenty different places. I have lived in Sheffield where I studied English at university, London, Chester, Shrewsbury to name but a few. I now live in Nottingham where I do the odd poetry gig; reading this stuff out. I love to paint and display my work in a cafe in Nottingham. I love the movies and have written a film called the naked ghost. I hope one day to write and direct my own film.

I have suffered with hearing voices since the age of twenty one. I also see visions and have been attacked by invisible forces such as snakes and spiders I have felt them crawling all over my body with no real explanation from the doctor just that I am ill. The voices in my head range from friends, to famous people to God or the universe as I call him, to strangers. Most of the time the voices are quite chatty and conversational other times they are very insulting and very repetitive. I've been sectioned under the mental health act four times for my own safety. I have learned to live with the voices and live quite a rich and full life.

This book of poems has taken me ten years to write, writing a poem every so often. There is a huge range of themes contained within this volume

Land of Ice

Camera on Diaz

Cameron Diaz will you marry me?

I'm fat, bald and short and have to pay for every escort.

Cameron Diaz will you marry me?

I can't dance or romance and tend to walk around in my underpants.

Cameron Diaz will you marry me?

I'm so ugly compared to you, but then who isn't?

Cameron Diaz will you marry me?

I wanted a life less ordinary, a life in all it's fullness, but then without you, all I got was life in all it's dullness.

Cameron Diaz will you marry me?

I can't stand the Trousersnakes' music. I've learnt more from chewing my nails. I'll sing to you, I'll sing out of key, I'll stand up in the pub and sing Karaoke.

Cameron Diaz will you marry me?

I've seen your beauty, I've seen your smile, I've seen that even when you're in your rags you always emanate style.

Cameron Diaz will you marry me?

I'll shave and bathe and never shop at Kwik save. I'll wash up, I'll vacuum and even tidy the bedroom.

A. Sole

Cameron Diaz will you marry me?

x x x x x x x x x x x x x x x x x x x x x x x x

Bull it sh

There was a man who made a machine.

With it, he thought, they'd make the planet clean.

Although, instead, they made it red and put a lot of innocent souls to bed.

The machine, they used, used a lot of lead.

However, I have used the lead to write a bunch of poems instead.

With the hope that, this lead, will help a lot of innocent souls get out of bled.

U.S Say….

Deliver banana peels to everyone's front door and someone's gonna slip up.

Drop bombs on a country and someone's gonna get their revenge.

Give a gun to everyone and someone's gonna get shot.

Drop bombs and one is gonna hit miss; the teacher of the class.

Wars over oil? Well the victims don't bleed the Texas tea as far eye can see.

U.S.A rules okay? Only when they make the rules up as they go along.

Their way!!!!!!!!!!!!!!!!!!!!

The Black Mamba

Mambo Mamba.
Come walk on by.
Mambo Mamba.
Look me in the eye.
Mambo Mamba.
I'll rise up six feet high.
Mambo Mamba.
I'll do a little dance.
Mambo mamba.
It'll put you in a trance.
Mambo Mamba.
This is no romance.

Mambo Mamba; the dance to the death.
Mambo Mamba: I'll take your last breath.

Mambo Mamba.
There's one thing I'll give.
Mambo Mamba.
One gift to leave you with.
Mambo Mamba.
It won't help you live.
Mambo Mamba.
For death is my game.
Mambo Mamba.
Life is my aim.
Mambo Mamba.
They'll never make me tame.

Mambo Mamba; the dance to the death.
Mambo Mamba; I'll take your last breath.

A. Sole

Mambo Mamba.
Mambo Mamba.
Mambo Mamba.
Mambo Mamba.

Land of Ice

Muhammad Dali

Sting like a butterfly.

Float like A bee.

Rumble art Rumble!

6 Billion Planet Earths

It's all in your head.

It's all in your head.

It's all in your head.

It's all in your head.

It's all in your head.

It's all in your head.

It's all in your head.

It's all in your head…
…and only gone when you're dead.

Land of Ice

The day I stood still

He came, they saw nothing and I stood still.
The fire in the briar means a lot to me.
I can speak to dog but does that mean that I'm barking.
I can see the wolf spirits and I can see them go.
In Devon the sun will smile on me,
And he shall burn with the embers of agony.

One two three four, hell is knocking at my door.
The Devil came round with a cigarette.
I gave him a light my fire and a funeral pyre
Sire, I said, isn't the situation just a bit too dire.
He replied, as he dried the cancer on his hands.
It's sympathy I seek and death is my demand.
So I said go to hell and tell them there;
There is no room for such ungodly despair.
Rare, he said, I like my meat
Especially when it's covered in Peat.
Oh yes now that would be a wondrous treat.

Oh but I think I'm barking up the wrong tree.
Maybe evolution, heaven and reincarnation is the key.
Maybe I just see what I see I see I see saw
On the sea shore I stood still and wondered;
Why is it so beautiful and what the hell is going on?!

A. Sole

The break

The sky about us.
The sky within me.

Sun, stars and clouds are all reluctant to leave.

Memory removed.
Memory released.
And memories escaped.

There are rhythms required to release the deceased.

Just deliver me from?
From whatever I fear.
From the words I fear.

As if my conscience should ever here appear to you my dear.

Goodbye Charlie Brown.
Don't drown alone.
Or worry about my tone

For me there are vast, intrepid and choral horizons.

Goodbye Charlie brown.
Don't drown alone.

I'll keep you always kept inside as I ride through new liaisons.

Goodbye Charlie Brown.

Always remember my heart will miss what my mind didn't want.

Land of Ice

The melancholy wanderer returns

I'm losing myself on a white sky day in January.
The sky layers itself, like my personality; very thinly.

Nobody and everybody hears the silence.
I see people's pursed or pouting lips.

Sound is now sent to me through machines.
Machines that sing or screech.

In the pubs and clubs talk is tamed.
Tamed, made lame and deranged.

Out in the street single mothers meet and greet.
Here the winds steals the sounds I need the most.

The sun splits, shakes and breaks my concentration.
Its divides me up into new emotions; a new sensation.

I'm slightly dulled or slightly honed but newly toned.
I'm a new man, not an old man with a new plan.

I abandoned lifeless suburbs where adults work their
daily roles.
Where children play with toys, trees and remote
controls.

I've roamed and wandered through this urban jungle.
I hiked and hitched through this country's little stitch.

I'm still so weary and wary and home is something so
scary.
I think I need a drink of normality from life's dairy.

It is really a shame I can't remember who my friends
are.

A. Sole

Friends made my life worth living before the adventures true misgiving.

It is really a shame that my past, present and future are all in my fizzled head.
I'll tell them a story but then they'll know it just something I've shared and shed.

Land of Ice

Her ingrained venom

What worries will I have in death?
Will it be the devils breath?

To be or not to be?
That was the mother fucking question.

To me, it's you must be and then must die.
You live, you die and in between you lie.

Maybe down?

I am invincible right now,
I'll be invincible tomorrow.

Life you're my bitch today
and you're my whore one tomorrow,
when it's time to pay up.

See then how she treats you,
when you're turning blue.

When you're looking through the looking glass,
and everything you know is past.

At the point when everything turns back and black.
Do blind men see the light at the end of the tunnel?

The end.

God's great big bit of nothing.

I always imagine the Earth in the true reality, size and ratio was a particle of dust.

A particle of dust floating through others heading towards that great coffee table in the sky.

I think this goes some way to explain why I rarely polish the place.

I mean its a terrible idea to think that I just Mr Sheened a galaxy away.

Even one that's surrounded by a few wine and coffee universe stains.

Land of Ice

Box of condoms

I knew from an early age that people;
friends and strangers would put me in a box.
I'd be this or I'd be that.
An opinion would be formed.

I knew at a later age my carcass would be put in a box.
Put in a box and then probably forgotten.

Although the box I forgot about was my so called home.
The dwelling that surrounds me, imprisons me and
dwells about me.

It's because of these boxes I decided to put myself in a
box
and mail myself to Thailand in search of sun, adventure
and hopefully some chicks, preferably without the dicks.

The remote control

The solemn silence
of a boring moment,
for a open heart,
on a blue evening
with a trapped freedom.
I believe I know now
why the caged bird sings;
because it's got fuck all to do
but make noise and eat.

Fill 'er up

This is the hollow world.
This is the stuffed world.

The mad scientists have sucked it all out.
The consumer junky has spat it all back in.

It was formed, spawned and sold to us all.
Next it was crushed, mushed and pushed back in.

We are the Junkyard dolls.
We are merchants of rubbish.

I've recycled my recycling.
Now it's all junk again.

We are the bean counter men
We are the has been men.
We are the bin men.

Hell, oh there

In the heart of darkness
I felt so cold and warm.

In the heart of darkness
I felt so bold and torn.

Where are you now?!
Where am I?

I'm in the heart darkness
and can smell it's sulphur breath.

Quietness, love, warmth and beauty
I wish I'd never known.

I'm in the heart of darkness
and have never felt so alone.

Land of Ice

The high burnt nations

The fallen leaves now dead are pavement wreaths.
And dark new days are drowned in doleful dreams.
This change in age reflects in me; I heave
my heart down darkened roads. I hear those streams
Of golden summer days where I last played.
There many sons dried up and scorched the land
And leaving Autumn winters timely raid.
No real escape by turning ticking sand.

These lands are low in salt and high in
cholesterol and toxic fumes that children mend.
They've caused such smoke to cover this my life.
They've pushed my heart with ease to cancerous strife
Then left me to walk in the present tense.
And wonder when this waste will finally end.

A. Sole

Voyager

I'm a traveller. My life's not dull.
Joy, safety and excitement are all eye know.
I'm always channelled into something full
and now a magic place where eye can go.

Eye no that eye know when I'm on a roll
and when Earth's my Oyster I'm learning to cook.
Eye will always watch you all score my goal
and know that eye was the one born into luck.

I've seen all the money and seen it burned.
My numbers are death, fourteen and the womb.
Gamble the gamble the space trips I've earned.
You can't lead me to face or fear my doom.

For with my fingers mortal precision
it's all mine on my television.

Land of Ice

The last rose

My house is next to the main road
cars pass by like multicoloured wasps.
It's the middle of the winter; January,
and snow's fallen lovingly on the ground.
In front of my home, my house, is a garden
and within that garden is mangled old rose bush.
A huge bush covered in snow both green and white
except for a single pinky red rose that is open and awake.
A thin layer of snow rests upon it's head and shoulders
so it droops slightly down, and it petals are frayed, old and frail.
But listen this rose is awake, alive and trying to go the distance.
None of the other roses are out to shout and show me what it's all about.
And dear rose, dear petals, dear pink and red, here's a note to say thank you.

R a i n clouds

I'll suffer the rain for the clouds,
 that paint pictures in the s k y.
I'll suffer the **night** for the *sunrise*
that awakens the newborn day.
And I'll suffer thepain to keep her love
<u>that shines through my *misty* grey life.</u>

Land of Ice

Hypothermiac

Life is so cold in this land of ice.
But you'll keep me warm.
You'll keep me warm.
Keep me warm.
Keep me warm.
Keep me warm.
And if I grow tired and fall asleep,
you'll know that I am dead.
Life is so cold in this land of ice.

A. Sole

Ex-stinks shunned

I turn a light on and we're one step closer to the end of
this planet.
I turn on a car and we're all gonna die.
Planet earth; welcome to the graveyard!
The graveyard, the graveyard.
Will you sell me the Capital when you can't see it
anymore?
Welcome to the smog. Welcome to the fog. Welcome to
the chemical weapons.
Please, gentlemen, do take your seats.

Imagine if I was alone.
Imagine if I was alone

.

Imagine If I was alone.

What will the last thing I see be?
A Chestnut tree?
An early morning sky?
My nearly mourning relatives cry?
Or just a cheery wave goodbye?
What will the last thing I see be, before I die?

And the rain screamed thunder, after the flash had gone
away.

Land of Ice

You night

Harm moany
Harm only me

You are breath of wind that has travelled around every temple, flower garden and all the perfume section in shops.

I am the breath of six in the morning after every fag, beer, curry and everyone of the poppadom pickles choices.

You are never ending beauty; exquisite in every sexual action that you gracefully do.

I have lost three teeth and can't stop farting in bed.

You are night.
I am dazed.

You are bright.
I am hazed.

You are night.
I am day.
Lets just live together
while we've got the bills to pay.

Work, rest and pray

Polishing flaws that don't need cleaning.
Settling scores that don't need meaning.
Dreaming dreams that don't need dreaming.

Hope is a rope.
Dope is a mope.
Coke is a smoke.
Screen is a mean.

Drive, drive, drive your car crazily down the street.
Crazily, crazily, crazily, crazily until you hear the heat.

Life happened in hours, minutes and seconds your honour.
It was all the now; the now and the now and the now and yes the now.

To eternal infinity and beyond.
But not beyond the grave.

Excuse me! If you are a lie, lie down over…
…there! Now if you are a clown am I a smile?
Is there such a thing as an everlasting green mile?

It has come to my attention that elevators go up and some might not even come down.
We must ban walking then.
Ha ha yes! That'll teach 'em.

Land of Ice

The mad house blues

Calypso won't let me go.
Medication is sick.
It don't make me tick.
I have a story to tell.
I have some ancient trees to fell.
I can smell the floor for miles.
Let me go.
I'll take the jacket with me and the magazine!!!!!!!!!!!!!!!

Love if...

Love is hoping to help with the belief that you'll receive.

Love is the belief that you'll help with the hope that you'll receive.

Love is you filling in the rest.

A. Sole

Diet Popular soft drinking and eating contest

New die tikka
New die ticker
New die terror.
New die terror
New die tame.
New die etiquette

But oh!

Give me a Penis

Give me a Eating disorder.

Give me a Prize.

Give a Sigh

Give me an Indignation.

And what do you get?!

Death and taxes.

Oops!

Opulence.
Oranges.
Pleasure.
Sex.

Oak.
Ornaments.
Pleasure
Sex.

Omens.
Orifices.
Pleasure.
Sex.

Orbits.
Oxygen.
Pleasure.
Sex.

Ooh!

Opulence.
Oranges.
Hate.

Oak.
Ornaments.
Hate.

Omens.
Orifices.
Hate.

Orbits.
Oxygen.
Hate.

Land of Ice

The human thing (Well that's what we've named ourselves)

How can it be, that I can be?
How can I be, the thing that I am?

The thing that I am is the um thing in the mirror.
I'm that things reflection. No that thing's a reflection of me.

Eyes, ears, nose, mouth, body, arms and legs and that sort of thing.
What else did I need?

A smile!
A tear.

I am water and stuff.
I am thirsty stuff.
Clever stuff.
Human stuff.

I'm a walking talking human thing.
Sorry what?!
What do you mean I'm gonna die some day?
Oh right. Well, as long as I get enough time to figure out what I am,
I'll be sound as a pound baby. I hope. I hope.

How can it be...

A. Sole

The nature of the night

Night intrudes my sleep when there's so much to do.
I found myself a brand new blue.
The night's awake, the night's alive.
Where the Werewolves duck and dive.

An electric light makes me feel so bright.
I feel relaxed and feel uptight.
The nights alive, the nights awake.
Will the moon thrust and quake the waters of an empty lake.

Look, at the end of road there's a squirmy little toad.
I know he hasn't read the green cross code. Zoooooom.
The nights alive, the nights awake.
The stars'll make the rivers bloodstream swerve and snake.

My footsteps across where the grass is glistening.
It's a hoot to know the owl is listening.
The night's alive, the nights awake
I hear the icy water falling break and grasp my spirit as I drink it straight.

The night's alive! The night awake.
Don't give me rocks or ice to break.
The spirit chills my blood to wake from this wondrous state.

For the days awake, the days alive.
The sun blasts the world with a forcefulness and drive.
Although it is the night that will always thrive with a beauty in my mind.

Morning Milkman can I buy a bottle of milk off yer?

Land of Ice

Hay days

In Hades today we're all insane.
Our dreams have all dried up.
We scorn on those who in their brain
do drink from a golden cup.
No fighting fears on life and death.
You know that dreams fall through.
Our sweats, our shakes, our icy breath.
Where do they fall in you!

Nowhere, for I've got my dreams,
and don't care for those who scorn and laugh.
For sunlight shines on all the streams
and mines a golden bath.
Cos I'll seize the day I'll seize the night.
I'll move and change and roam.
I'll take my dreams into the light
and make a happy home,

A. Sole

On English weather

I was on a train and it didn't rain.
Got off the train and I got wet.
And I'll take a five to one bet that the clouds will swarm
and the rain will storm the moment you leave your
brolley at home.

Land of Ice

Lost in a prison

I knelt down at the edge of the Atlantic ocean.
My knees sank slightly into the sand.
The moon echoed in the water.
I gazed ever so unsure of what lay before me.
Did I ever exist, do I know??
I have memories, a tiny multitude of short film scripts, all in Technicolor.
Memories like northern lights flutter around my brain?
"It's a goal!!!!!! Ronaldo scores for united. Lovely goal that Brian..."
Huh. Oh the televisions on.

Depressing play

With muse and music I live and love that sound, that sense of play.
Play? Meaning; Engage in games or other activities for enjoyment rather than for a serious or practical purpose.
Play? Meaning to have fun in a game.
Life could be a game?
I'd hope so, if I didn't know so damn well it wasn't.
Bollocks.
Play music, that's a serious and practical purpose.
Couldn't live without it.
I hear music playing all the time.
Life's still not a game.
Music: sometimes I relate, sometimes I hate.
Sometimes I love and it makes me live.
So lets face the music and play.
Play.
Play but don't get played.
Play my song.
Play our song.
Play it again sample.

Land of Ice

Just trying to get me some peace

So in that test tube is a virus so deadly it would kill 99%
of the population of the planet?
Yes that's right.
And you've found out I'm one of the ones immune to it?
Yes that's right.
Can I hold it?
Sure, but don't drop it.
Oh, oopsy daisy.
Oh dear God!

A. Sole

The writer's block of sand

Fly over the desert with me now, the vast, vacuous and vacant desert.
See, amidst the desert, the wordy, worldly writer is sat at his dirty, dusty, desk.
Here, upon his desk, is where the type is righted and the candle stands alighted.

Do you want to see him sighting all that his inner vision has invited?
Do you want to see all that his inner soul has ignited?

Hmm, okay, well let us stall and come to a crawl as we now trawl through the writers mind.
Let's peel the rind that covers the mind and unbind the acidic blinds to his windows.
We might even see the way he sees the salty seas that surround this desert's shore.
The artist's eyes are kaleidoscopic, he sees in, broadband, H.D, technicoloured truth.
I hope that you believe me, and won't leave me, because I have no other proof.
'I'm empty! I'm empty!' the artist cries, 'I'm empty and full and didn't know a world could be so rich and be so awful dull.'
'I just see a field, a sea of beings just waiting and waiting for the cull! But I'll tell you this; I once felt bliss in a single kiss and that kind of love is forever and ever hard to dismiss. But, now, go from here, have another beer and have no fear until death approaches you with a silver spear, ha ha ha ha ha, goodbye.'
Well then, we'll fly from this writer and hope he is a fighter or his world gets a little lighter, so his outlook will become a little brighter...

...tap, tap, tap, tap, tap, tap, tap, tap, tap, tap, tap, tap.

Land of Ice

Lazy, lazy give me your answer true. I'm half crazy...

I awoke from my death.
It was the morn.
My room was alive; lit up by a yellow effervescent hue.
Yeah, dawn's new sunlight shone seemingly through the dusty window pane.
I was awake, for the first time, I was awake!
Although, my dream were still hovering like haze over golden ocean waves.
I rose, through rolling waves of sheets, like Poseidon from the bottom of the sea.
As I did, I saw that a pen and paper lay on my wooden chest, my breast.
So, as I rose, I threw them down to the bottom of the briny sea of socks and junk.
My eye's soon filled with salty tears as I went back to the business of dreamz z z.

Enviro-mental

My house is next to a thunderous, thoughtless, pipping and parking main road.
The road has traffic lights, traffic fights, road perks and road works.
It's January, and there is snow.
I never sit in the front garden because of terrific amount of terrible traffic.
The front garden is my own freeway to the front door, nothing more.
Today, however, I saw something so plush that it made me blush.
I saw a Rose bush amid the snowy mush.
On that bush I saw a single solitary red Rose.
It was red, red like a Shakespearean simile for red.
The traffic hummed, chummed and shummed by without seeing my snowy January Rose.
My Rose buddy, surrounded in snow, please be there tomorrow to put on another show.

What do we do when the oil runs out?
What do we do when the oil runs out?
What do we do when the oil runs out?
What is really fucked?

Please My dear Rose don't disappear like a Snowman in the night.

Land of Ice

Poem E150d

The waves and spray splash my face as I leave the sand of my island behind.

The cogs turn and spin as my legs furiously pump the chained up peddles of my silver steed.

Clouds smother my vision, of the blue skies, in mist.

A soft breeze is there to tease my soul as it passes over the Atlantic.

Dolphins smile and mermaids wave as I spy the American Shore.

Now, first, in the U.S of A I go to business and Rodeo grind the Golden state bridge.

I bunny hop over the Empire state building in a single bound while breaking the speed of sound.

I one handed fake-manual the motorways from East to West and yet still I'm never blessed.

Again I take, take to the skies and to my surprise the people laugh and stare.

As if this gift was there's to share.

So I go somewhere else to find a place where people have more hopes in there mind...

'Babe, turn over, I fucking hate the adverts.'

'Alright, but put the kettle on will yer?'

Putting it into perspective

I'm in a 3D world
with 3D rain and
3D puddles.

We have 3D pain.

In a 3D world
we can go anywhere.

We have 3D happiness.

In a 3D world
there's always cubes
and never squares.

We 3D have sadness.

In a 3D world
I can look up and
look down.

We have 3D madness.

In a 3D world
the sounds surrounds
me.

We have 3D fear.

In a 3D world I'm
always surrounded
without a 3D escape.

Land of Ice

Our roots

Tearing down trees just to see the root.
Tearing down trees just to pick the fruit.
Tearing down trees to get a full magazine.
Tearing down trees just to play with matches.
Tearing down trees just to make or break some homes.
Tearing down trees now you see the age.

If you take something give it back.

I see a tree clinging on to a leaf for dear life
like a man clinging to his wife for dear strife.

I see a tree not moving but our air it's still making.
Is there a tree on the moon?
Is there a tree on any other planet or star we can see?
I never hug trees.
But I can sit below them and hug the one I love.

How many trees does it take to be noticed that too many
trees have died?

I'm not a lumberjack and I'm not okay.
I do wear ladies underwear but I don't want to go into
that right now.

Poem X & why?

I live therefore I am.

I hope therefore I am.

I dream therefore I am.

I believe therefore I am.

I love therefore I am.

I trust therefore I am.

I die for there I am.

Land of Ice

Pole cats

The pole is not the soul,
But the girl that's wrapped around it
And the crowd that surround it.

Dance girl dance!

It's a ballet.
It's a soiree into muscle and moves,
Music and grooves...

Dance girl dance!

Applaud people applaud.
Let all the wine be poured.
Let all the ladies of the pole forever be adored.

I lonely I

My girl smells of perfume.
With my eyes closed I can tell when she enters the room.
In a naked garden she makes flowers bloom.

My girl's a poem.
My girl's a play.
My girl makes me glad that I'm not gay.

My girl's smile is always in style.
My girl's eyes always have spies.
And my girl's laugh never ever dies.

Land of Ice

Sixty weapons of mass destruction

The mushroom clouds my mind.
I just don't know what I'll find.

It's an explosion of colour and life,
With everything hanging on the button of a knife.

You're all dead.
You're all wed.
You haven't seen what you've bled.

Hallucinate.
Copulate.
Meditate.
Aim your hate.
Force everything to become a western state.

Yee Ha!

A. Sole

St Ikea

Ikea, Ikea, I fear Ikea.
Are we all the same?
Are the Swedish to blame?

Is my life flat pack?
Do these tables sometimes attack?

Have a hotdog and a Lot fwog table.
Was I put together to be so stable?

I'm going to saw a tree!
Maybe then I'll be free.

Ikea, Ikea could we be any freer
And any more dull and insincere?

So buy, buy and find a goodbye!
Watch all the other designers sigh and cry.

Land of Ice

The human race

The man who was born in the bronze age
Always looked best when he was on the stage.

The man who was born with the silver genes
Surpassed all the others who were on the scene.

But the man who was born in a golden shower
Found that he was born with enormous power.

A. Sole

My exist stance

Monsters, monster everywhere!

I keep seeing my own death.
I keep seeing my own breath.

I know we're all driving to the car park of Eden.
I've seen so many swimming in solid ice.
I know we're all paying such a price.

I keep hearing my own death.
I keep hearing my own breath.

Love and law are blind.
I am an orange without a rind.
I am a human but of a different kind.
I know you're killing me but I don't mind.

I keep feeling my own death.
I keep feeling my own breath.

Monsters, monsters everywhere...

Buy products

Faith is just a by-product of life.

Life is just a by-product of love.

Love is a by-product of God.

God is a by-product of beauty.

Beauty is a by-product of products.

Duality

I am Batman.
I am Clark Kent.
I am the Policeman that's truly bent.

I am the sky.
I am true love.
I am the bird that's sent from above.

I am the devil.
I am the God.
I'm just the poor sod that trapped in between
Like you I'm a being that's just stepped on the seen.

Kill and create. Kill and create,
Or just see what goes on when it gets late.

Land of Ice

Casing the planet

From the bottom of my heart
Right up to the top
I know I'm more than just a pretty prop.
I've got a mind and don't need to be signed.

Hell, I'm pissed in ecstasy!
Heaven, I've found a new tranquillity.

I've found the doorway it's down life's hallway.

I've got beaches and trees.
I've got peaches and seas.

I am the sicker man than a suicidal plan.
I know the end and have seen it bend.

I am the whale.
Now here me wail!!!!!!!!!!!!!!!!!!!!!!!!!!!!!!!!!!!!!!

I am the quicker man than those sperms that failed,
On a sicker planet than those that sailed.

A. Sole

Sold soul planet Sole

God wanked and Eve was created.
God drank and was inebriated.
God sighed and Mary smiled.
God cried and out came a child.

Microwaves, micro ways and holidays.
A place in the sun a spider has spun.
We got chicken and cheese but the vegetable has won!

I order food.
I order you.
I order mood.
I order glue.

Let's stick together.
Let's fall apart.
Let's clone a liver.
Let's clone a heart.

My name is not yours.
My father was a million whores.
My mother a chain of showroom stores.

The true Milky way is dead,
We opted for evolution instead.

I'm going to rest my head,
in my sleepy bed.
Now in my dreams
I'll hear the familiar screams
of the junkyard dog
who licked that very special frog.

Rib it, rib it and rib it organ.

Land of Ice

The marsh mellow man

And here he lies,
below the mist and below the skies.
In the muddy marsh the mellow man lies.

Forever he'll be lying in the marsh
and never will his body see the harsh light of day.
Never more can this man pray.
He's no more awake than when he was asleep.
No woman lying next to him. No women did weep.
Not even the one that kept his keep.

I know that one day his bones will turn to rock.
His brains will go all gooey like a Dali clock.
His body will turn to oil or just join in with the soil.
But I know it's a crime the cops will never foil.

My bullet's the only jewellery he'll wear.
I'm just glad I had one to spare.
I grabbed my shovel. I grabbed my spade.
Through the marshes I had to wade.

Now, I just have to say one last thing;
Don't shag my wife or you'll feel my sting!!

Body parts of the poem

My life is like a series of daydreams
Where nothing is as it seems.

My head is like an aeroplane
I don't know whether I'm high or just insane.

My heart is like a puddle
It's all wet and in need of a cuddle.

My body is like a cyborg kettle
With my hot soul encased within the metal.

My love is like super glue
And if you want it, it will always stick with you.

Land of Ice

Surf and turf

My computer has a glitch
It's like a whining howling bitch.
And now I won't get on to my C.G.I pitch
And none of my pixel players will get a stitch.

I have to reboot my system or it's
So I can look at the girls with the super size tits
And see if my pages have had any hits
And then change my brain into megabits.

I think therefore it is

We travelled to the moon in a thought bubble.
We flew through the air in a thought bubble.
We travelled under the sea in thought bubble.
We spoke from box to box in a thought bubble.
The thin king, the thinking!
The thin king is sin king.
We decided not to care in a thought bubble.
We blew up cities from the air in a thought bubble.
We shot people down in a thought bubble.
We made people slaves in a thought bubble.

Eureka, eureka this missiles got a seeker.

Land of Ice

Mother written on his arm

I met a boy who was born with tattoos.
He didn't say how many needles his mother used.
He did say she used them when she got the blues
And it was always the heroine she abused.

He said she said the needle set her free,
Aware that she was going to be trapped with a baby.
But then he said the only needle the doctor could see
Was the one that was sticking out of her belly.

A. Sole

Trampy's song

Trampy's just asleep in bed
So many souls; so many dead.
I'm talking through my open head.
Listening to the words that aren't spoken.

Maybe hope.
Maybe dreams
Maybe sunset.
Maybe screams.

Ba-ba-ba-ba -bah!

Tell you about my rubber heart.
Tell you about my brand new start.
The echoes pass; the echoes start.
I love that boy they pulled apart!

Maybe hope.
Maybe dreams.
Maybe sunset.
Maybe screams.

Ba-ba-ba-ba-bah!

I scream into the dirty wind that blow's so very cold.
I think about the icy grave
and know that I was never the one to be a slave
Just a slave to madness but never badness,
I smile again!

So maybe hope!
So maybe dreams!
So maybe sunsets!
So maybe screams!

Land of Ice

Ba-ba-ba-ba-bah!

But Trampy's just asleep in bed!
So many soul's; so many dead!
I'm talking through my open head!
Listening to the words that aren't spoken!
Ba-ba-ba-ba-ba-ba-ba-ba-bah

The windy and windy road

Carefully I rode the winding path
Through the forests on a giraffe
And just tried to have a merry old laugh
Cos the giraffe could see the winding path.

Yet since I've been mad
They think that I'm bad.
Yet since I've been mad
They think that I'm bad!
Yet since I've been sad
They've think that I'm glad!
Now tell me who's mad
if you think I'm glad?

I carefully listen to the wind!
I know it surely hasn't sinned!
And if it's sinned it should be binned
But then there'll be a lot of rubbish everywhere!
The wind has not sinned
And I am like the wind!!!!
Shhhhhh
Well for I am like the breeze
Who yes nurse will go to bed with ease...

Yet since I've been mad
They think that I'm bad.
Yet since I've been sad
They think that I'm glad.
Now tell me who's mad
If you that I'm glad?

The coach
The boat,
A woman with two children,
tears rolling down her mascara face;

Land of Ice

A mother,
A parent,
Alone with two children
one sleeping comfortably in her warm arms.
The dark sea.
A stormy sea.
A dull yellow light covering the room like a sheet,
as the ship gently rocks the tired cradle to sleep.
A lone boy.
A plastic seat.
The smell of salt, fags and alcohol drift through the air.
An unused cigarette rolling melancholy across the floor.
A trip?
A journey.
Sickly orange fizzy pop and a red and white straw.
A snotty nose, an untied shoelace showing my credentials.
Where's my father?
Where's my dad?
He always came along; to Cyprus, Paris and Japan.
Not this time, no, he was at home with the fights and the shouts.
Those tears then.
These tears today,
The tears as the moon lies restlessly on the Oceans skin.
And memories still flash by like an old silent film.
This lonely sea front.
This rocky beach.
These cool winds and the ships that pass from one shore to another
Like divorce papers passing from the one lawyer to the other.
Where's my father?!
Where's my dad?
The shrill of the wind the only reply, as my tears now slowly dry.

A. Sole

And I now again begin to cry as the stars shining they slowly die.

Land of Ice

Righting

A vacant moment stands me in good stead
As I think of all the books that I have read.
The chilling tale of how she lost her heart.
The chilling tale of how she lost the part.
Well I lost the plot or gave it away.
I made my mind just dance and sway, oooh!

Freedom of the mind is what I sought;
It's a funny old path as long as you don't get caught!
Freedom I need you like the sunshine…
Freedom I need you like the air!

The plot not taken is taken all again,
As I type for monkeys and other men.
Suckin' on a peach that's just out of reach
As I hope my words will reach and teach.
Chasing down memories in my mind,
Wondering what nightmare that I might find.

Poetry is in motion
And your eyes have just moved x x x x

Children of the weird ones

We're all ghosts within the dream.
We're all hosts that hold the scheme.
We're all happy in between.
We're all loved when we are seen.

Oh we're all chain smokers
And we're all pawn brokers
Yeah we're all sane jokers
And we're all pain soakers;
yeah yeah yeah!

Well we're all insane depending on who you ask!
I don't think that's a very hard thing to grasp; yeah yeah!
We're all in the rain whether trailer or trash!
I think we're all in the brain but I'll have to ask.
I know we all feel pain but that won't last, yeah yeah
yeah!

Can I announce myself to you?
My name is death
And I'm coming for you!

Land of Ice

Star fazing

Endless gazing at the stars,
Now I'm feeling like the king of hearts.
Always running through the clouds
Made me feel so awesome proud.
My head is ploughing through the waves
Made me remember all that purple haze.

Show me your love Earth
Make me live my second birth.
Oh I'm just sailing safely on the surf
Don't show me rubbish on the turf.

Sounds of Jupiter died again
Made me feel like I was ten.
Rings of Saturn round my head
Made my mind feel just like lead,
Oh my legs felt just like open wings
And my heart felt full of golden springs

Why doesn't Earth spin beneath my feet?
Why is everything so really neat?
We almost manage the tidy land;
This planet could have just been sand.
So really I just demand an explanation.

Wacko?

It's dark now and I go outside for a cigarette,
a man sit's on a wall, near girls.
I notice him straight away, as he wears a blue Trilby hat
And a light faded blue pin stripe suit.
I pay only a moments glance, I'm too busy, I light my cigarette,
While my mind rolls in work and out
To the dark street lit sky and black leafless trees, solitary stars.
The man, though, in the corner of my eye
Stands up and approaches me. Yet on his way softly swoops down
And picks up a flat, stubbed out fag end;
Crushed by a multitude of feet that have all gone to safe houses, safe homes.
He lights the smoke and then speaks to me:
'Have you passed?' Passed I ask. 'Yes passed, I passed... he begins to mumble.
Alone the uncomfortable confronts my heart
as it now begins to pound. Why is he here? So, why are you here? 'I walked!' he says
with a smile, with sparkly dull eyes, that suggest all
my ignorance, my folly and his pride for accomplishing such a task like that.
I slowly step back in realization. The girls laugh,
on the wall, in the distance, as they chat away, he laughs with them, not at them,
though not even I can hear them talk and I
am young, and he is old, sixty by looks; clean shaven, shirt and suit, well ironed,
tie straight, too straight, his shoes clean, shiny,
yet soles' rims caked in mud. Mud on the bottom of his trousers from feet
that have walked too far, too closely together.

Land of Ice

My heart beats; faster now. What is this strange instinct of fear that's
awakening me? I stare at him. He stares
into the distance, into nowhere, bends down, stubs the cigarette end
out and picks up another and lights it,
Then walks away, not away; around, mills around. I put out my cigarette,
and go inside, away, and call security.

Why no

I shouldn't have got drunk, last night.
I shouldn't have got drunk, last night.
I shouldn't have got drunk, last night.
I shouldn't have got drunk, last night.

I should have got drunk, last night!
I should have got drunk, last night!
I should have got drunk, last night!
I should have got drunk, last night!

The life lottery

I'm rich!!!!
I'm rich, rich, rich!
I'm richer than my wildest dreams!
I'm so very fucking rich!!
Now all I need is some money….

Land of Ice

Heaven is a place for madmen

Sanity why are you such a profanity?
Eagles swirl from the sky down on my invisible mind.
This is rat country I think you'll find.
See them terrorize dawn's sunlit parade
with their chemical tirade.
Chemicals mix with chemicals
to form my altered state of consciousness.
I am the drugged up man with a drugged up plan.
I am the chemicals that pulsate around my brain.
Oh the right chemical at the right time
can show heaven what it's missing.
But I am the injection. The depot man, the chemical man!
The mind controls my body clocking in and out Nutzville.
Yes tomorrow sir I'll be as fine as a line on a page_____
But today sir I am a scribble
but please don't quibble the mental health is all I have....

Tuesday at six o clock in the morning I stare out the window.
Who is that person and where does he go so slow.
Birds don't sing to me, don't talk to me either.
I close the window and close my soul.
The room is filled with Guy Fawkes' cigarette smoke;
A line of Coke, a line of Coke; I think I'll soak in a line of Coke.
No thanks, no weed this time for there is no reason and rhyme
That would help me find the time to feel so sick and so unwell
Hell is where the weed lies burning just like the devil's tail.

A. Sole

I've never felt so destroyed as when I smoke the Weedy
Ganj!
So a Line of Coke will take my mind into today,
Oh say can you hear me? Will you be near me when I
die?
Ahhhhhhhhhhhhhhh yes now I'm ready, now I'm steady
Go!!!!!

Sleep deprivation is the song of the nation.
It's a new sensation,
just when the parties over turn out the night.
'Sole I got to get going man.'
said a reveller in the art of the hardcore.
But my dear Buzz man
there is no Fuzz man
and the shop opens in half an hour.
Flower Power is a tower we all have to climb,
I think as Love plays on the machine.
'Sole the goal of the party is accomplished
our minds have gone in one and that's the rub!'
The man in the white straight suit leaves.
I sit and wonder what he really believes.
My eyes tear the room apart as they slice
through the cans and cups and Cocaine.
The hallucinogenic screen, the trippy television screams
light and colour.
What's that God? I ask the voice in my head!
'The party is over and the end has just begun.
 I think you need to see what's in the Sun.'
God, the universe, whatever you name is,
 game is, shame is, let me go.
I don't want to hear voices any more!!!!
'But my dear sir' says the devil,
'what would you do without me?'
 Oh I see, well I'd just be
 and see if some girl would marry me.

Land of Ice

As I loom my naked girl enters the bloom
of the silvery smoke of the front room.
'Sole, I'm not dressed!'
'Are you sexually repressed?'
Don't get stressed
put on a vest and marry me.
'Ha ha oh Sole are you staring at my mole?'
'You were when I was sliding down the pole.'
No your mole is blind and so am I
to your imperfections of a kind.
'Well you can't be true'
'you've got too many voices other than you!'
Well sunrise to sunset,
I know sometimes I'm quite a good bet.
'I don't play the gambling game,
'and it's a shame that you can't be tame!'
Oh but the wild man in me is the pussy cat in you!
'Well you'll have to let the cat out of the bag...'
'..And get in here for a damn good shag!'

I lie next to her
and see her purr
as the smoke begins to stir.
We ride like Hunter on a motorbike
wondering where the edge is.
Humanity is sexual conflict and war
and all the other things I abhor.
But she is so beautiful
it's just a shame she's not dutiful, any more.
Our bodies become one;
two devils coming for you.
'Well,' says the devil, 'sex and drugs and Rock n roll'
'might just fill the hole.'
So will evolution,
I think it's the solution
to getting you out of my head.
'You're better off dead!

A. Sole

'You're better off dead!'
'Sole fill my hole.' She says
 as if she heard what the devil said.
'And it's not my goal to kill'
'you're open soul with the marriage lead.'
'I want to set you free'
'and see you roam and party'
'like you have no home.'
 Babe I respect you like I respect God
 with an open mind and a little nod.
'There is no god Sole'
'it's only a voice'
'just love me like you have no choice!'
 It's a voice!
 A voice that won't leave
 and has many stories that it must weave!
'Well this tale must fail before I marry you'
 'and lead life that's merrily just for two.'

I'm sober,
I'm drunk
with Cocaine up my trunk,
I leave and take a shower.
The fair maiden in bed
had gone to my head
and is covered in red, white and blue.
If she's true
I know that we are through
and that's why I'm so unwed, white and blue.
She attacked me first with such a burst,
that I didn't know the force of my own power.
I threw her off the bed
and she hit her head and for a moment
I thought that she be dead.
She howls in the bedroom that I beat her up.
I just tell her to shut the fuck up!
She wails on the bathroom door

Land of Ice

as if I wanted more from the psycho girl that I adore.
The scratches on my face
will leave a trace of the empty place I found my girl.
I mean I merely said she put on some weight
and hope it wasn't a baby in the crate!
'Sole, you bastard!'
'Get the hell out here now so I can kick you.'
'So I can show how,'
'How I go to town on the clown that broke my nose!'
'All ready for my dancing Shows'
She starts to weep and I keep washing my bone
as they feel like stones buried in the earth.
You know I love that girl for all she's worth
and maybe shouldn't have brought up the birth.
Death is always the end
and shouldn't be mixed with the start,
I broke her heart.

Honey, I'm sorry, my priceless party princess,
who I love from recesses of my darkened mind.
'Let me inside so I can see the divide'
'and the damage you've caused between us.'
I get out the shower;
I cower behind the door
as I see my flower covered in red white and blue.
You're in a mess, but please don't stress, just get
cleaned up and put on a nice dress. Yes?
'Sole you hurt my soul,'
'but now I only have one goal'
'and that's to get showered and get changed.'
Well I'm glad to see you're less deranged, I made a
mistake
that you'll just have to forgive and forsake.
'Well you're lucky its not you that I forsake,'
'but now I have my hair to wash and rake.'
Women!
Will you I ever understand how they can, on demand,

scream hell then whisper heaven.
Since I was eleven they made me shine
and made me fine and made me see the woman divine.
Since I was twelve they made me delve in deepest darkest parts
of my heart when they start to depart.
I love you girl and will never leave or deceive
and marriage is only a false conceit designed to defeat.

The Kitchen looks like Lord Kitchener wanted you there last night!
But not this morning, I start to sing like the King.
A party executive is asleep against the wall;
a bottle of champagne is the only sign that he's had a ball.
I make a cup of coffee. I have three sugars and drink it black
now that's when the voices begin to attack.
'So we're a woman beater are we?' says the devil in my head,
'I wonder if she'd look better off dead?'
I'm no woman beater, it was self defence,
dear voice in my head,
I merely pushed her off the bed.
'You know what the neighbours will say;'
'that you were her prey,'
'when they see it in the light of day.'
Well it's lucky I don't care what the neighbours think,
 even if they really do want to raise a stink!
'Just think tomorrow, all over town,'
'you'll be the druggy boyfriend that beats up his girl!'
'Don't worry,' says God to me,
'you know the truth will put those gossip in a twirl'
Go from here the pair of you!
This head is designed just for me and not for you too!
Is that not true?

Land of Ice

In the front room, I notices, it's become a drunken tomb
for a girl that's passed out behind the couch.
I slouch into the couch and feel a right grouch,
the voices have fell from the pouch that's in my brain.
I'm crazy and will have to deal with it; the shit.
I live in two worlds while only walking in one.
You'll all see the world around me the Coke with the host
but you'll never hear the voice of a ghost.
Demon's come to stay, while my friends all like to play.
Film stars come to speak any day of the week.
I've seen visions of heaven and visions of hell.
I've heard and I've seen things that I could never tell.
I light a cigarette, a Marlboro light and watch the smoke rise in the light.
Don't worry about all this shite!
A woman walks passed the window and I give her a smile.
She puts me on trial. Good morning!!

I have another line from the mirror that's made me blind
and sometimes so unkind and less defined.
I'm an orange rind a soft centre is hard to find,
but with a wooosh I'm feeling stooosh and more refined.
I think I'll put some music on, a bit of the Clash
and always avoid the Hash as it stares at me on the table.
I fought the law and the law won.
Sectioned four times but I'm still smiling.
I fought the law and the law? Saved me?
The worst things about being committed;
you are crazy, it all gets hazy and the drugs make you lazy.
There's nothing to do, but eat, smoke
and get a poke in bum by the straight jacket drug.
What a bug to bear, but I don't care
cos these are high times and I'm feeling fine!!!

A. Sole

Time to shine like that sun is through my dirty window pane.
God I wish I was sane.
'You're one of the greatest men on this planet,'
'and I'd never question your sanity.'
Thanks but that coming from a voice in my head is mere vanity.
My mind made it up. See?

'Sweetie, are you alright? I'm sorry about the fight.
 Let's not make it ruin such a lovely night.'
Oh god, look at your face. I feel such a disgrace.
I shouldn't have thrown you about the place.
'Well it does look bad, but then your scratches'
'are just patches of the pain I felt.'
Well people are gonna think I beat you down
in the heat of the rounds of shouts and screams.
'Well we are a pair that's to be fair'
'and the people around here don't scare me as they gossip and see.'
Well I am really sorry and you are not to worry
 that will never happen again, oh man I love you Jen.
'Kill her!' says the devil, 'Kill her!'
'Cut her wrists with the razor blade and you'll be forever made.'
'I love you too Sole, you are my only goal'
'oh except for that and the pole that I truly love.'
You were sent from above my silver lining,
my true gold mining made for wining and dining.

I'll sing that I'm you're broken king
if you'll be my sticky glue queen?
'I'll sing that you're the greatest king'
'this crazy old world has ever seen!'
Love you bruised girl!
'Love you scratched man!'

Land of Ice

I am the chemical man.
I am the drug man.
I am the drug, man.
Insanity is a profanity that I have to handle.
So just burn for me a little candle.
Or just send me straight to heaven, straight from hell x x
x x x

A. Sole

Cross the streams

The night was dark. The boy was pissed and bored.

Notice the rocks that look like men.
The silent leaves; too wet to rustle.

I wake, Oxygen, like a wave,
Blasts through my aching body.

Let's nail plastic, porcelain, wooden,
white, cold Christs to our golden silver walls.

I feel the surf waiting for me.
I hear the spirited shifting sands.
It's all calling, falling through the wind chimes

Ketamine is tranquillity in a broken glass.

One day I'll be free from concrete.
One day you'll be free from me.

I'm laughing at the man in the mirror.
I'm asking him to strange his ways.

Ellie's eating Skittles in bed;
They're the grapes for the modern generation.

The ugly are the bitter race?!

I'm drifting on a highway made of glue.
It a road that's never made for two

The moments of pleasure and pain
are just there to stoke the embers
of sadness and madness and joy.

Land of Ice

Being alone only becomes loneliness
when it's interrupted by other people.

A. Sole

Survival of the fittest?

These people are dead!
Crushed by a world
That neither liked them,
Loved them or needed them.

They walk alone,
Or in small groups
Like stagnant puddles
Cast out by the main stream.
The stream that trickles
Down drains.

To hear them is to hear
Nothing and everything.
For fear has crushed and mushed
Their broken souls.
And bruised hearts
Tell a very beaten tail.

A hot poker through the heart;
will kill a gentle sole.
A violent whip across the soul
Will shatter a weaker spirit!

Cross off your peace with love.
And let love be you
And let you be loved x

Land of Ice

Maxwell's demon

The darkness in life is all in my head:
It's the eye I see when I go to bed.
It's the ghosts I see when I'm off the meds.
It's the blood I see it's all the reds!

Voices, voices echo and blast!
I hope my future is not my past.
Voices, voices echo and blast!
I hope the die hasn't already been cast.

I see the darkness it's in the light.
I hope my brain doesn't turn to night.
I hope my fight is always right;
To see me well, to see me bright!

Delusion: An idiosyncratic belief
Or impression
That is not in accordance
With a generally accepted reality...

I've been stabbed with invisible swords
And invisible words.
I've slept in a bed of invisible spiders
And snakes.

God do you hear my cry?!
Will I scream your name
The day that I die!!

Believe in God and you're so sane!
There's nothing wrong with your holy brain.

Here his voice and you have no choice
Than to be shored at a mental health ward.

A. Sole

Believe in ghosts and you're quite hazy.
See a ghost and you're quite crazy!

There's no such thing as ghosts!
It's all in the head.
There's no such thing as god!!!
Except when you're dead!

Is the Devil all in the mind?
Or has Science made men blind?
An answer to this I've tried to find.

But stand in your churches!
Stand in your labs!
See if there's a medal up for grabs.

Was it the voices in his head
That lead Jesus to being dead?
Joan of Arc and Socrates
Give me an answer, if you please.

What if five add five doesn't equal ten?
What if the clocks don't all match Big Ben?

My name is A. Sole I've been sectioned,
been committed four times.
I've spoken to demons.
I've spoken to God.
I believe in love!!
I have seen hate.
I tried to kill myself
to see if there is a golden gate.
But for now you'll keep me warm in this land of ice.
And if I grow tired and fall asleep
you'll know that I've gone to find out.

www.ingramcontent.com/pod-product-compliance
Lightning Source LLC
Chambersburg PA
CBHW022205080426
42734CB00006B/558